T0380902

Written by Clementine Marianna Joy

MEAGLE SAYZ

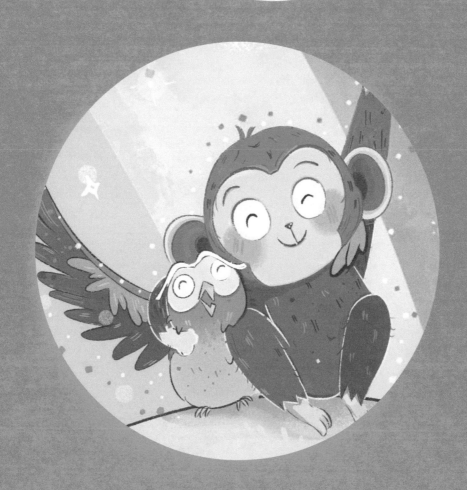

Illustrated by Funti

Archway Publishing books may be ordered through booksellers or by contacting:

Archway Publishing
1663 Liberty Drive
Bloomington, IN 47403
www.archwaypublishing.com
844-669-3957

ISBN: 978-1-6657-6275-5 (sc)
ISBN: 978-1-6657-6276-2 (e)

Library of Congress Control Number: 2024913528

Print information available on the last page.

Archway Publishing rev. date: 07/09/2024

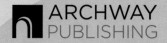

Dedication

To my brother Nathanael, whose giggles,
love, and affection have made me understand
the reality of life of a special needs child.

Context of the story

Meagle is a small brown monkey who has special needs . He has a special talent for noticing things. Meagle discovers that he is different from other monkeys. He faces challenges that the other monkeys do not, such as being bothered by loud noises and changes in routine, which can overwhelm him at times. Meagle goes to his role model and best friend, Piko, an old and wise owl who lives in a cozy tree hollow. Meagle seeks Piko's advice when facing challenges. Piko is patient and understanding and helps Meagle understand his feelings and learn about the world around him.

In a vibrant jungle filled with life, a young brown monkey named Meagle lived.
He felt everything around him different.
Sounds were louder, lights were brighter and changes were hard.

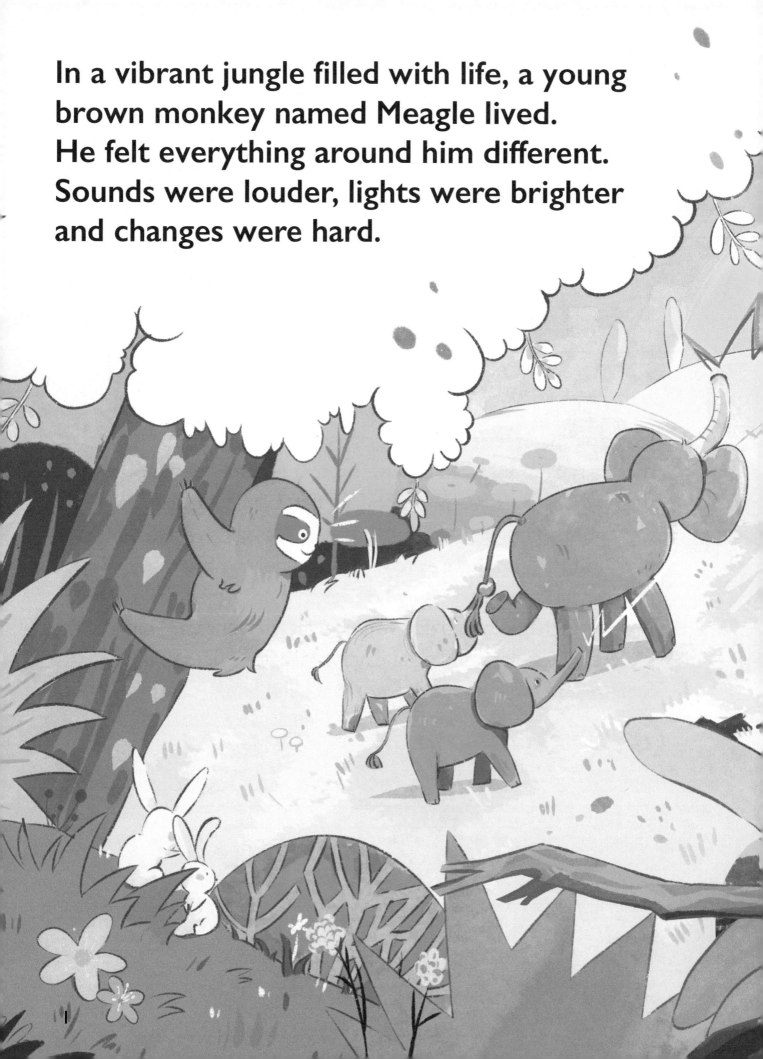

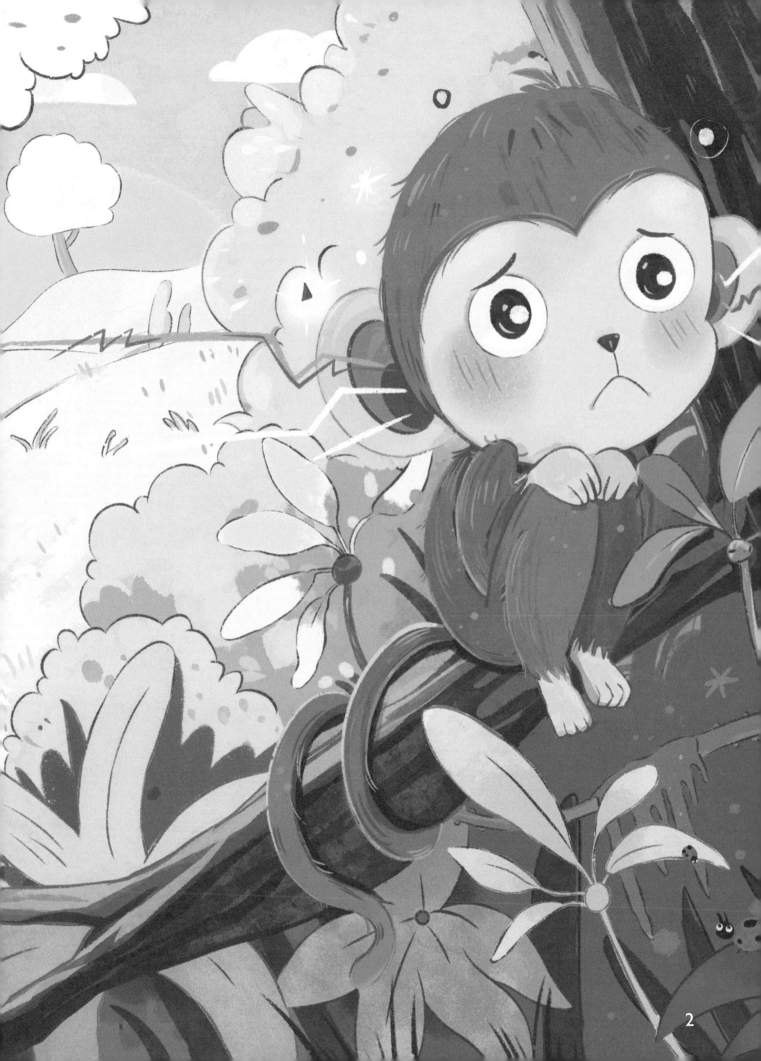

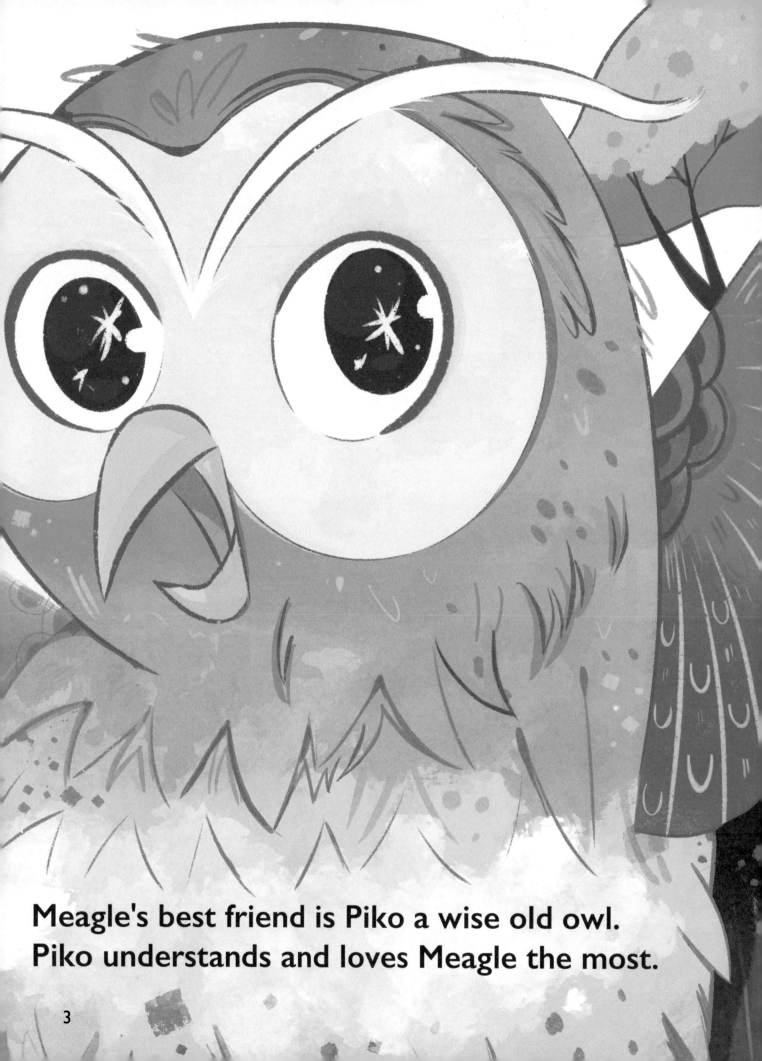

Meagle's best friend is Piko a wise old owl.
Piko understands and loves Meagle the most.

One day, Meagle ran to Piko and said

"OOOH OOOH AAH OUCH"

"What happened Meagle?" Piko asked.

Meagle said, "The jungle is so loud,
Meagle ears hurt."

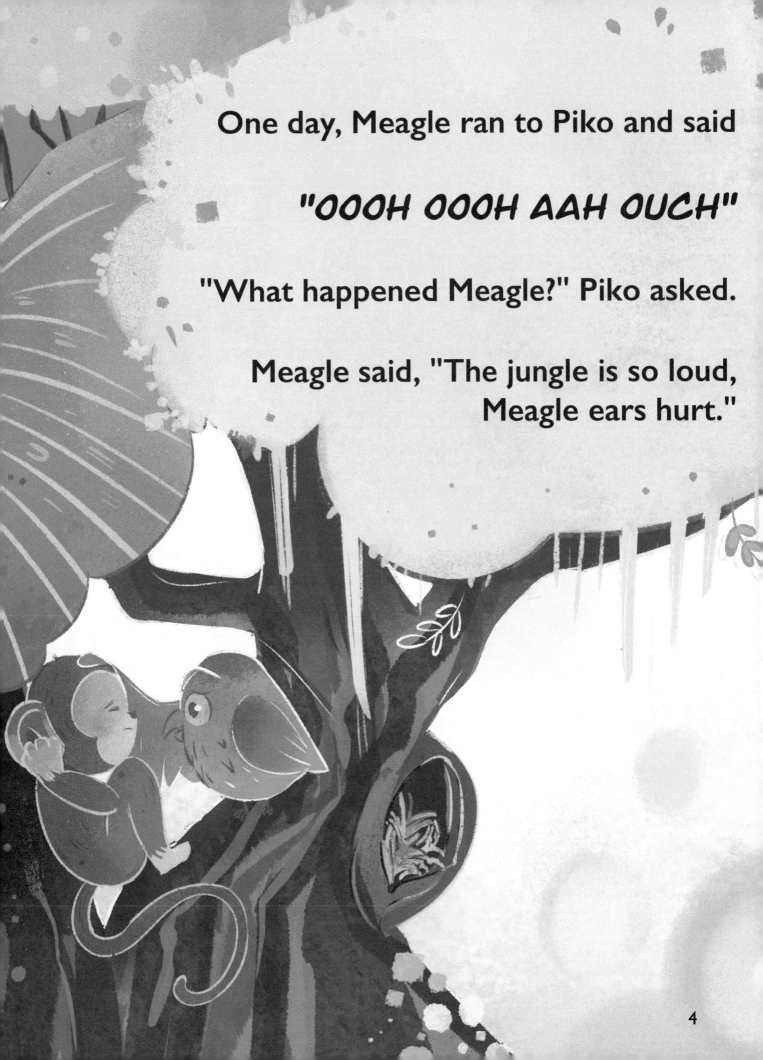

Piko looked at Meagle and said
"Everyone is different Meagle and
you have special ears. You could hear sounds
that many of us cannot."

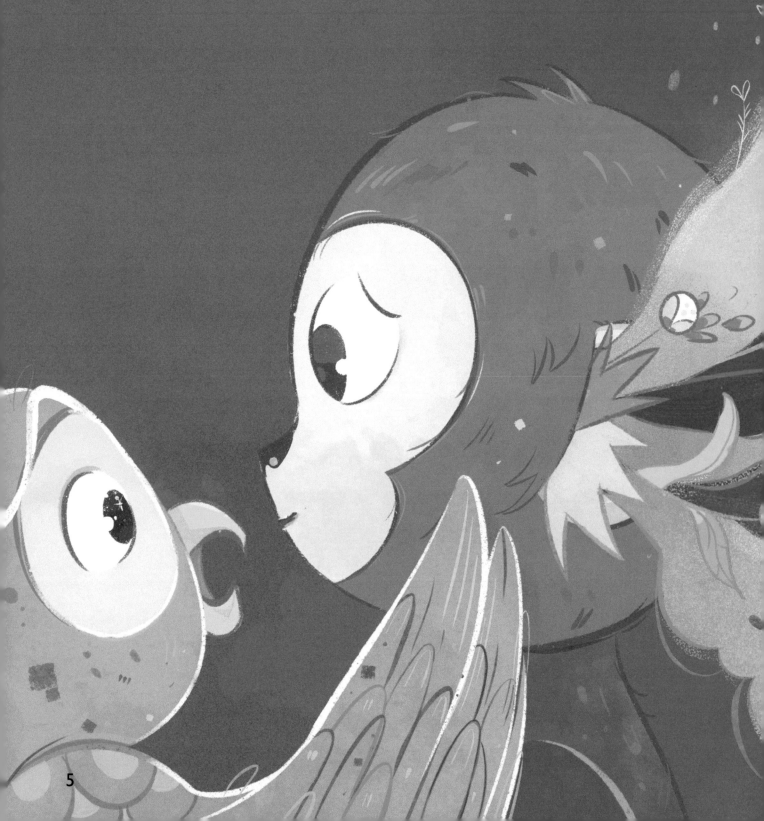

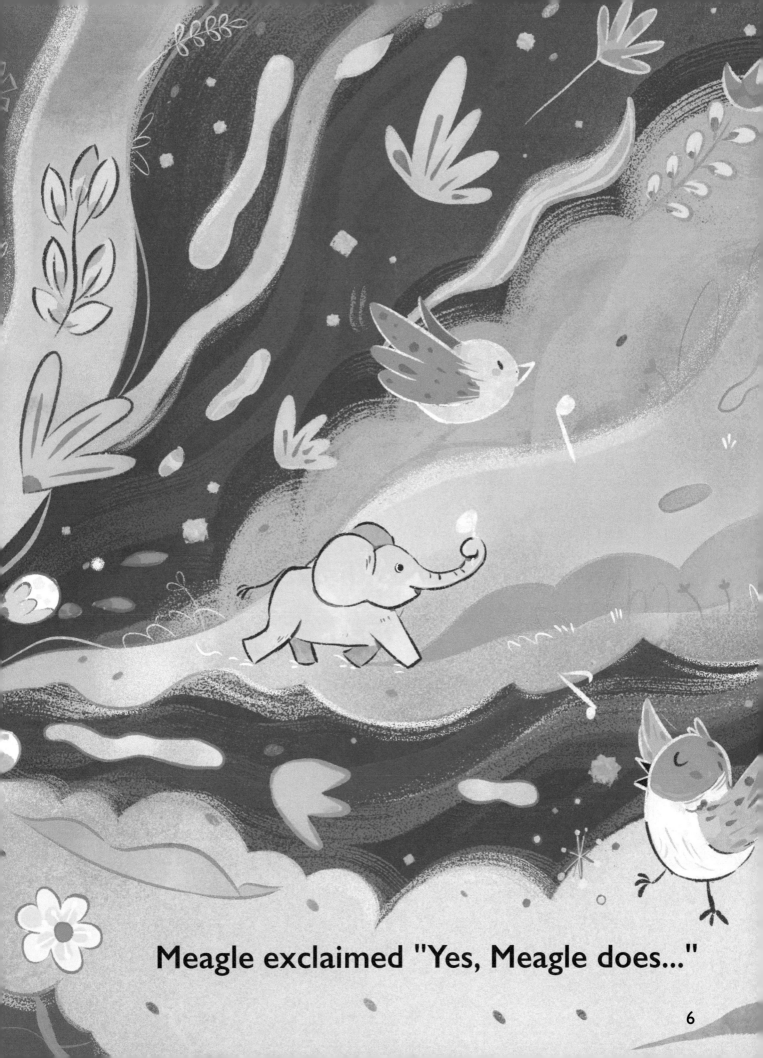

Meagle exclaimed "Yes, Meagle does..."

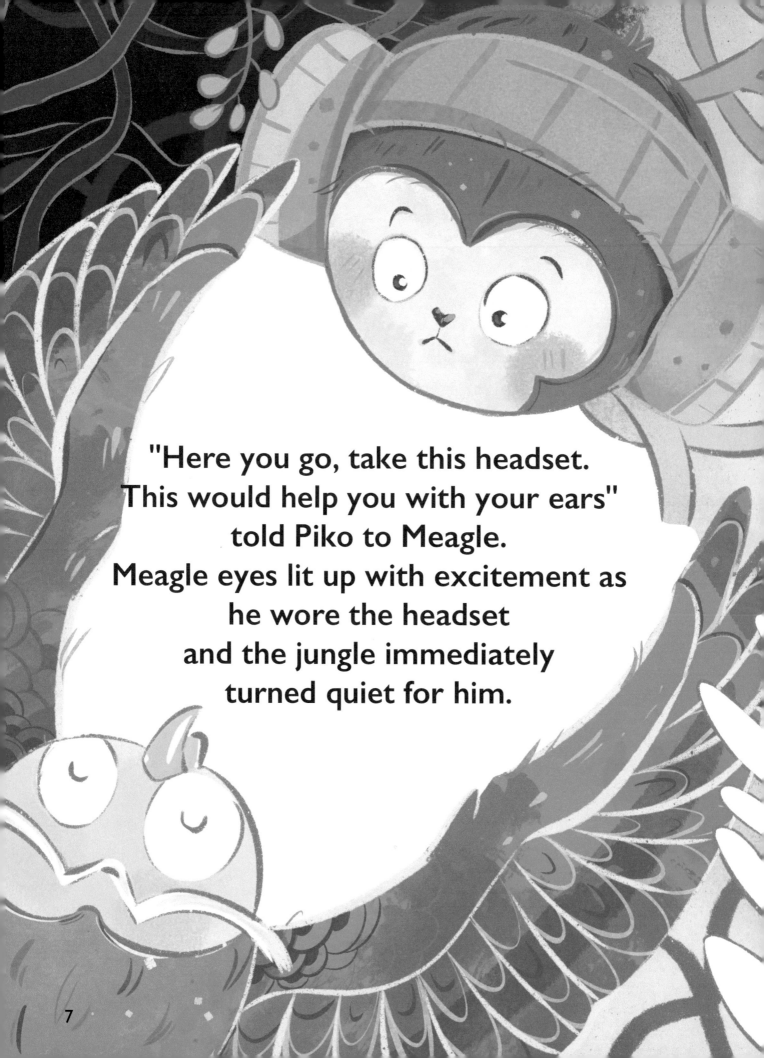

"Here you go, take this headset.
This would help you with your ears"
told Piko to Meagle.
Meagle eyes lit up with excitement as
he wore the headset
and the jungle immediately
turned quiet for him.

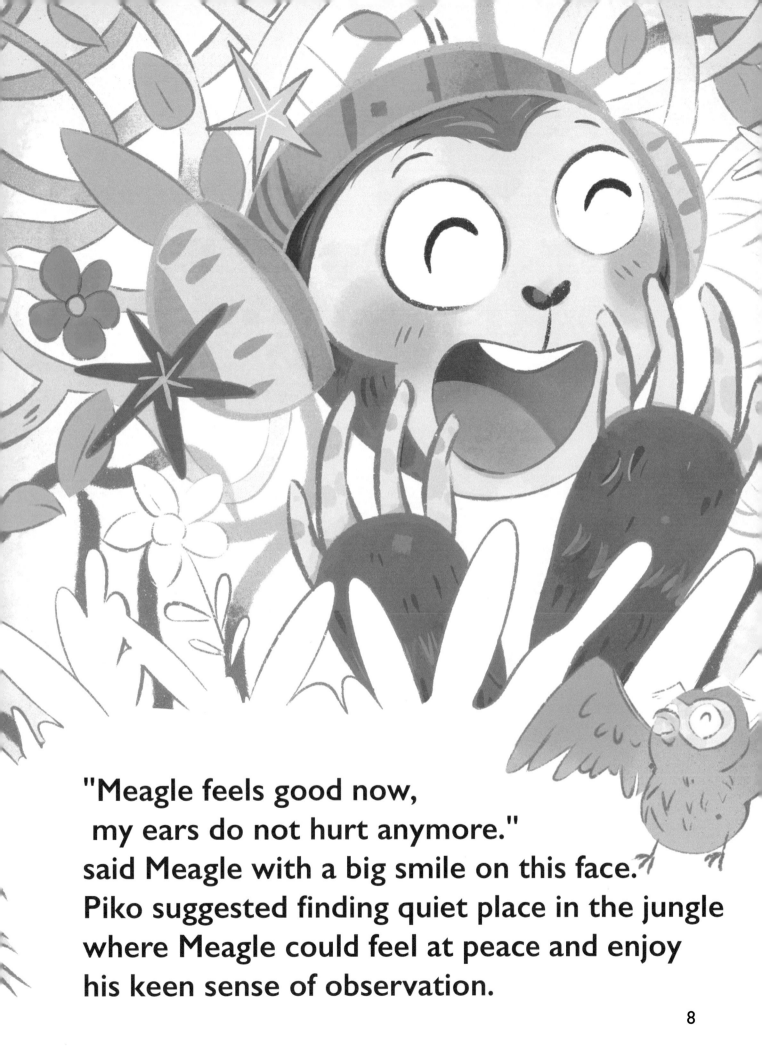

"Meagle feels good now,
my ears do not hurt anymore."
said Meagle with a big smile on this face.
Piko suggested finding quiet place in the jungle
where Meagle could feel at peace and enjoy
his keen sense of observation.

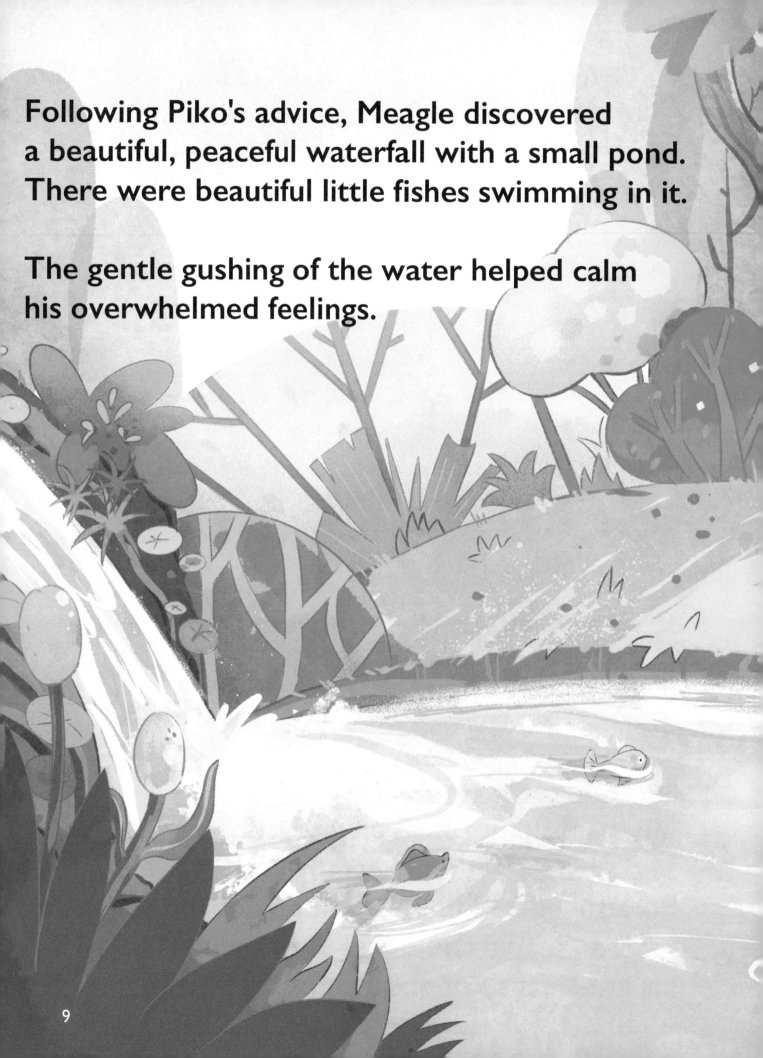

Following Piko's advice, Meagle discovered
a beautiful, peaceful waterfall with a small pond.
There were beautiful little fishes swimming in it.

The gentle gushing of the water helped calm
his overwhelmed feelings.

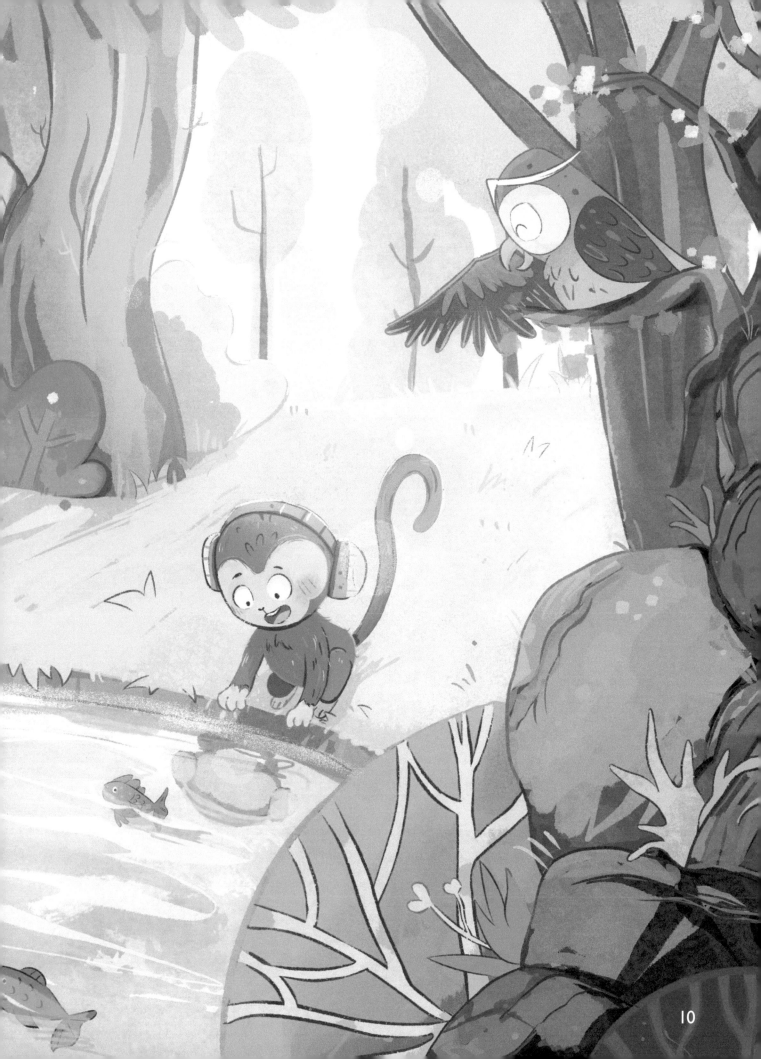

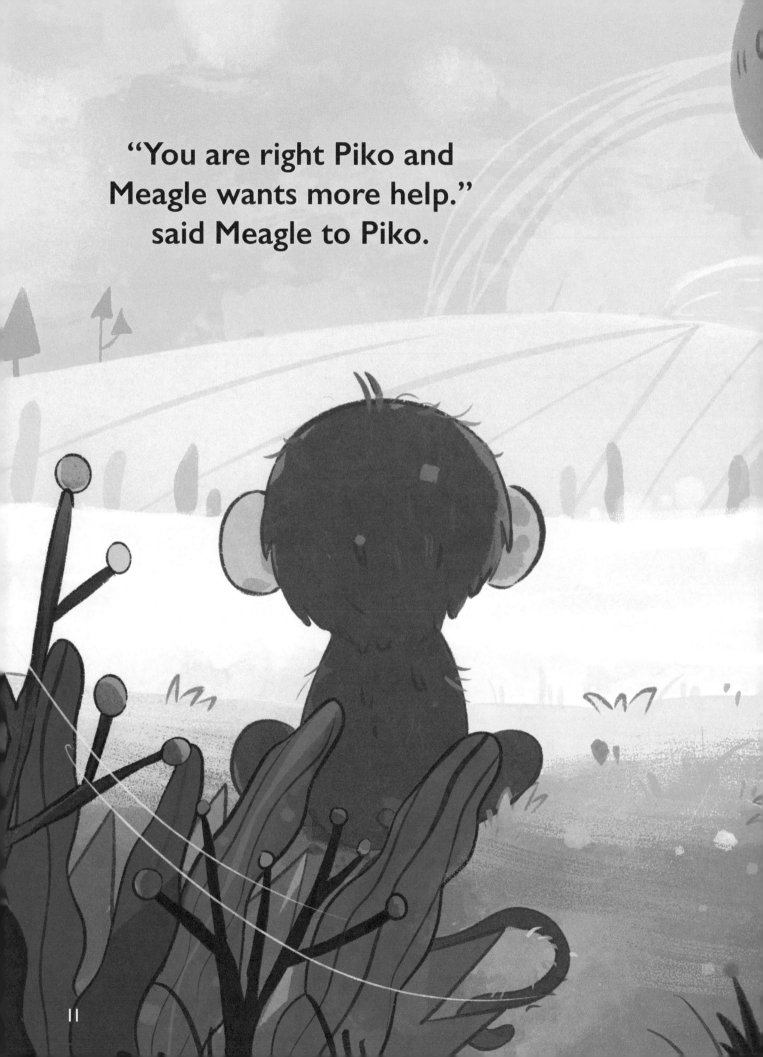

"You are right Piko and
Meagle wants more help."
said Meagle to Piko.

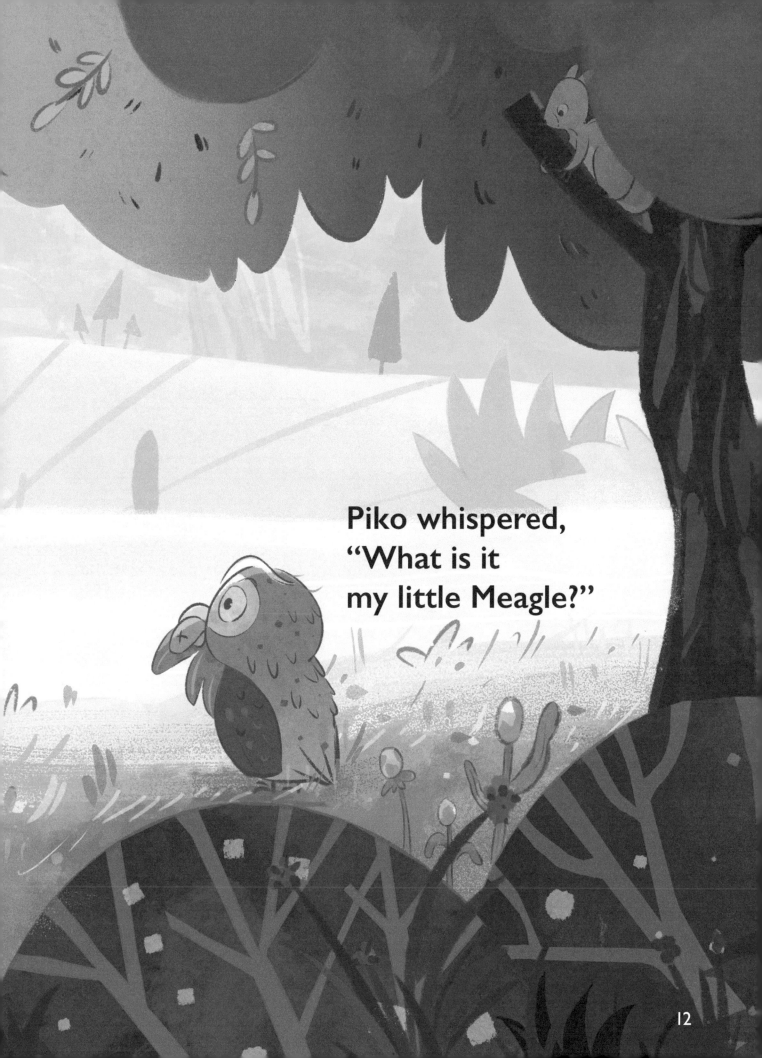

Piko whispered,
"What is it
my little Meagle?"

"I have a lot of toys and I love to arrange them in a straight line. I also want everything in order" whispered Meagle.

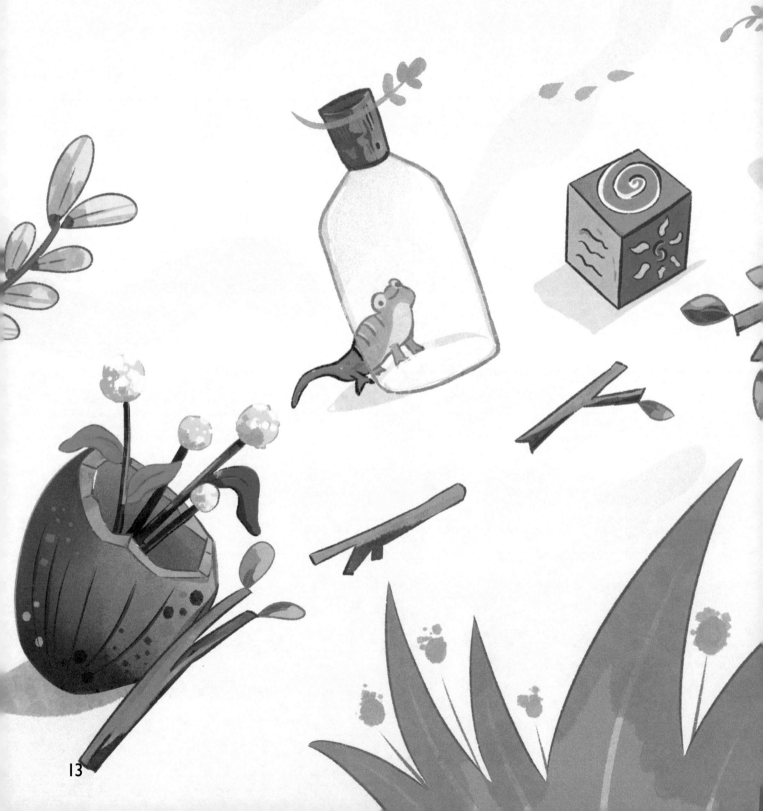

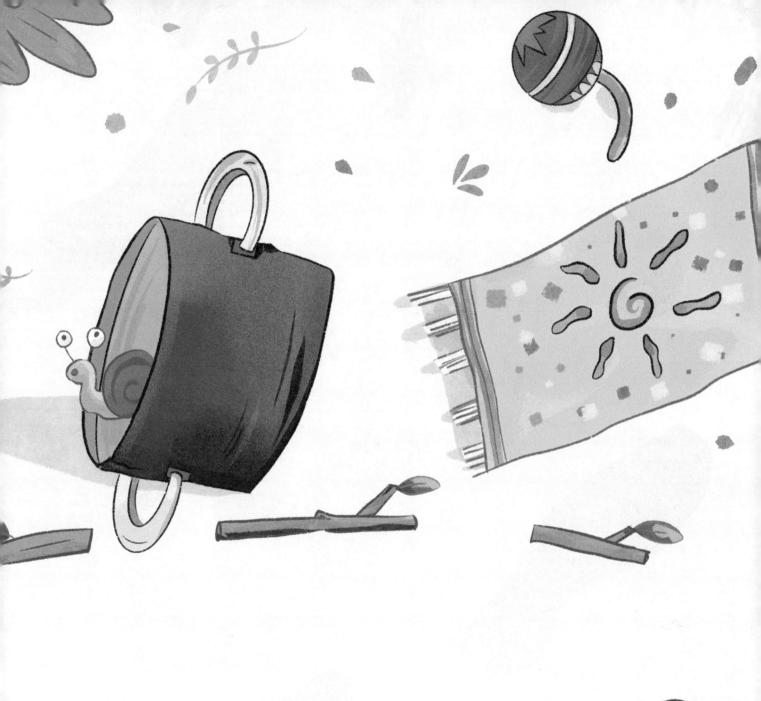

"Hmmmm, that is not wrong. Everybody loves to play with their toys differently and you love to keep all your things in the place they need to be." replied Piko.

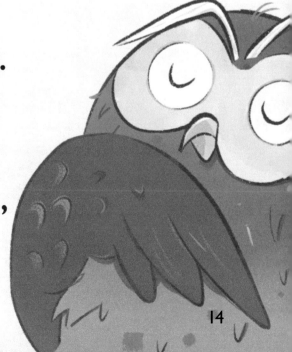

With an innocent voice Meagle murmured "Meagle also does not know when other animals are happy or sad!"

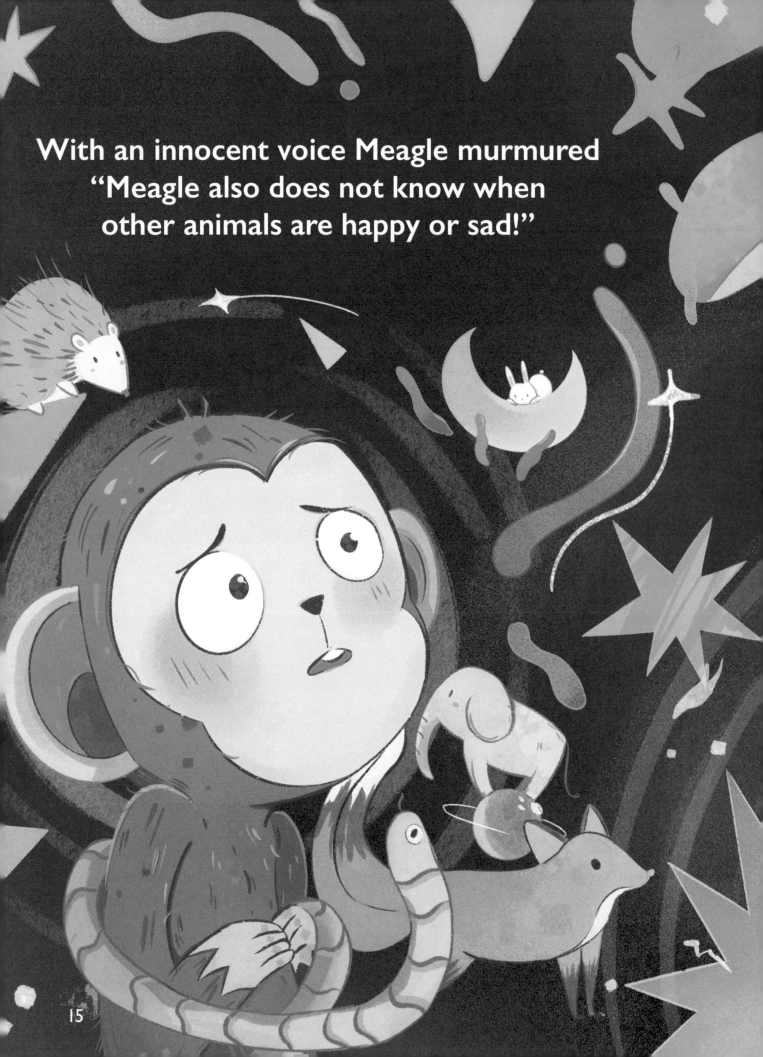

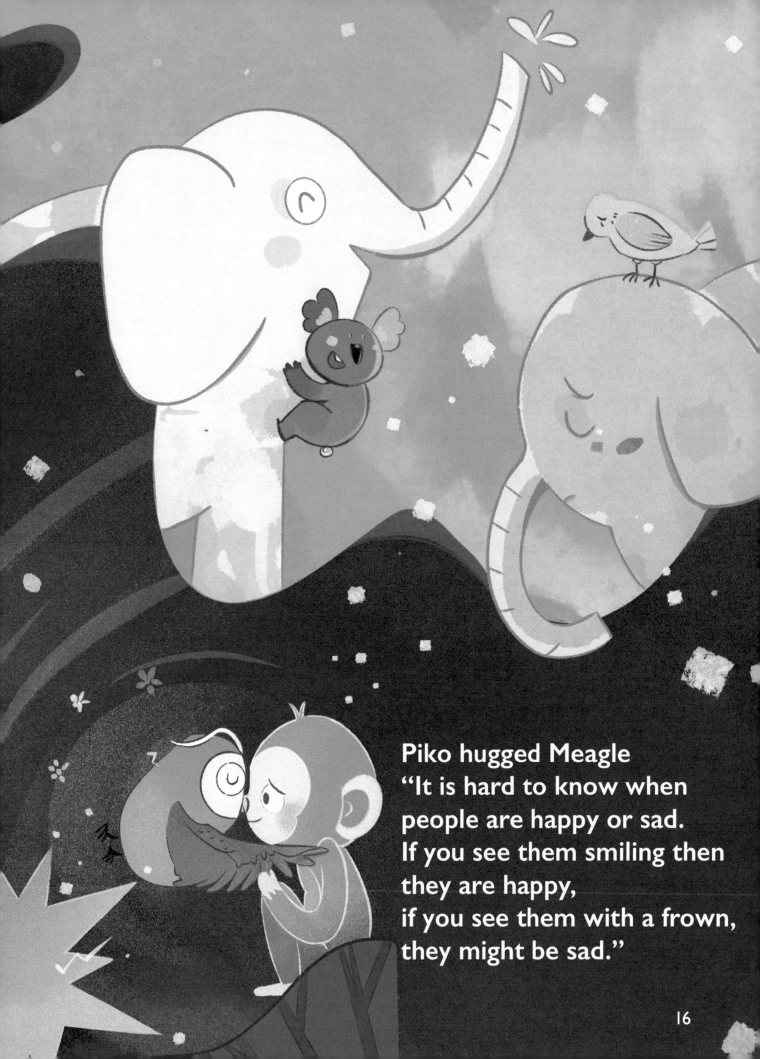

Piko hugged Meagle
"It is hard to know when
people are happy or sad.
If you see them smiling then
they are happy,
if you see them with a frown,
they might be sad."

16

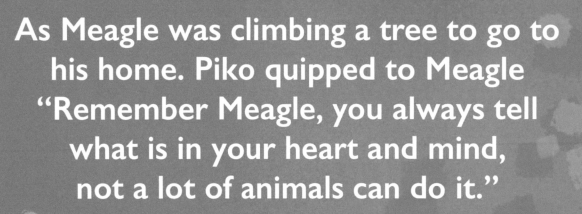

As Meagle was climbing a tree to go to his home. Piko quipped to Meagle "Remember Meagle, you always tell what is in your heart and mind, not a lot of animals can do it."

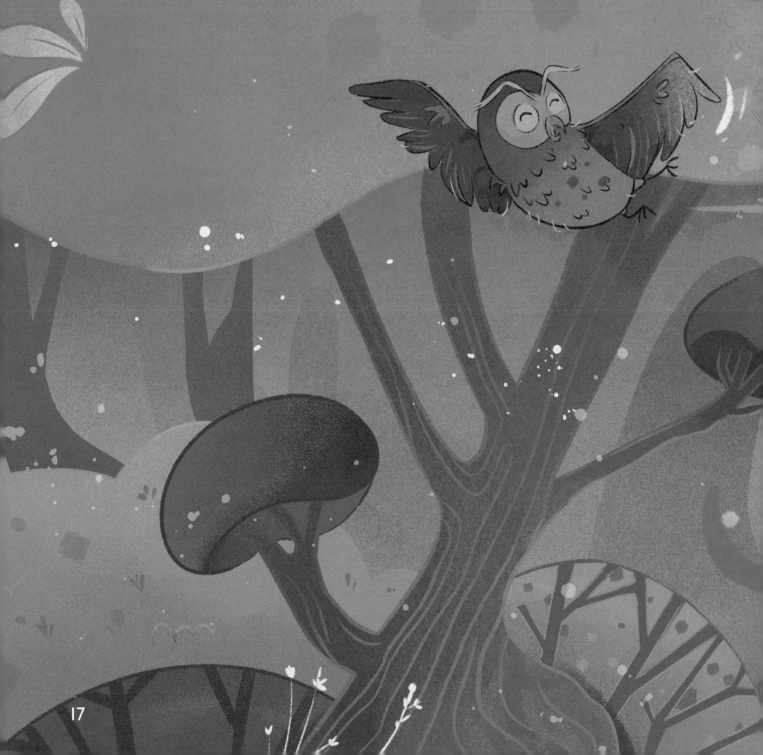

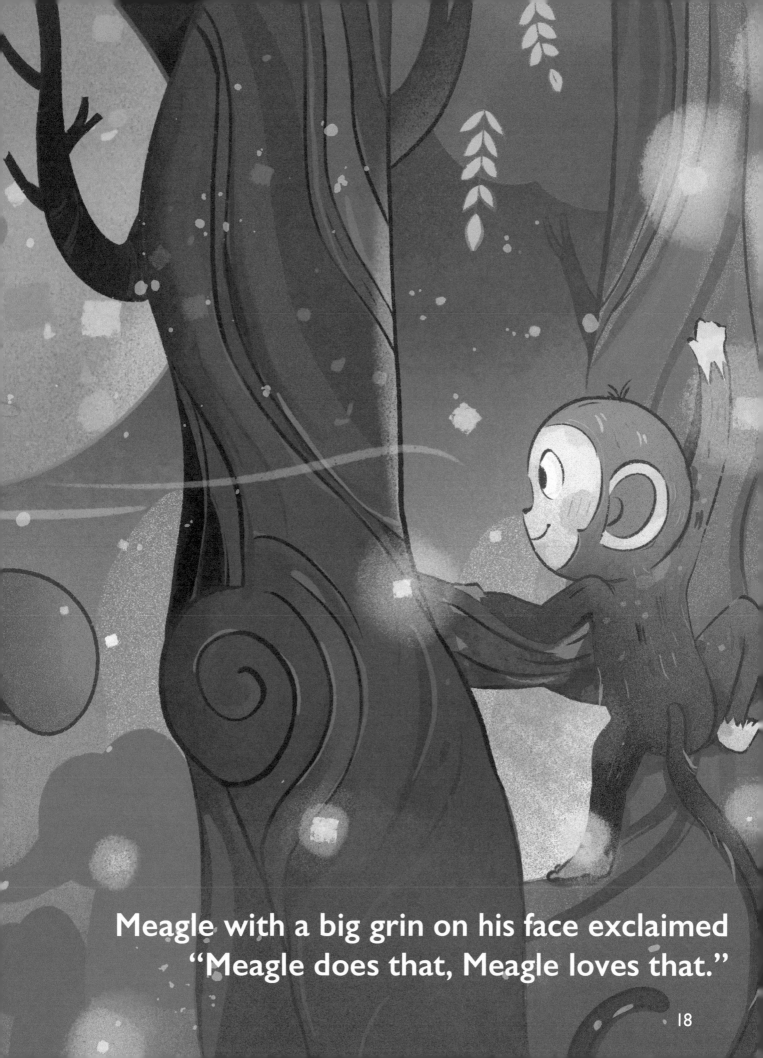

Meagle with a big grin on his face exclaimed "Meagle does that, Meagle loves that."

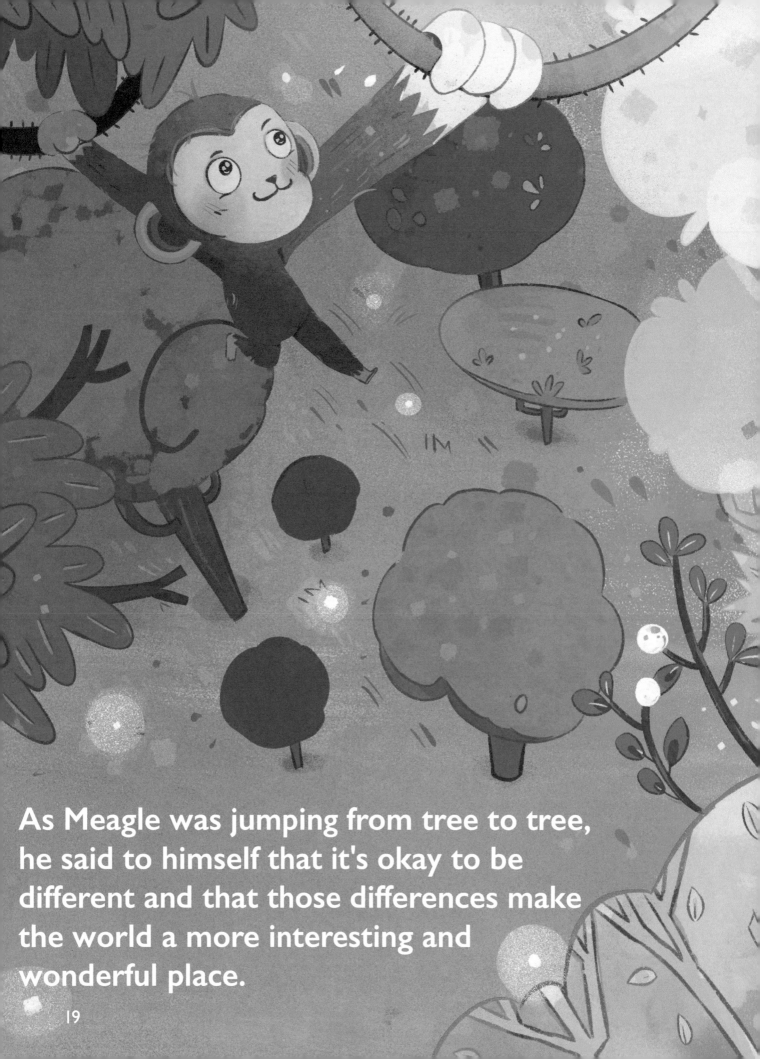

As Meagle was jumping from tree to tree, he said to himself that it's okay to be different and that those differences make the world a more interesting and wonderful place.

Embracing his uniqueness,
Meagle became friends with
all the animals in the jungle and became
a beloved member of the jungle family,
cherished and loved
for his special talent and kind heart.

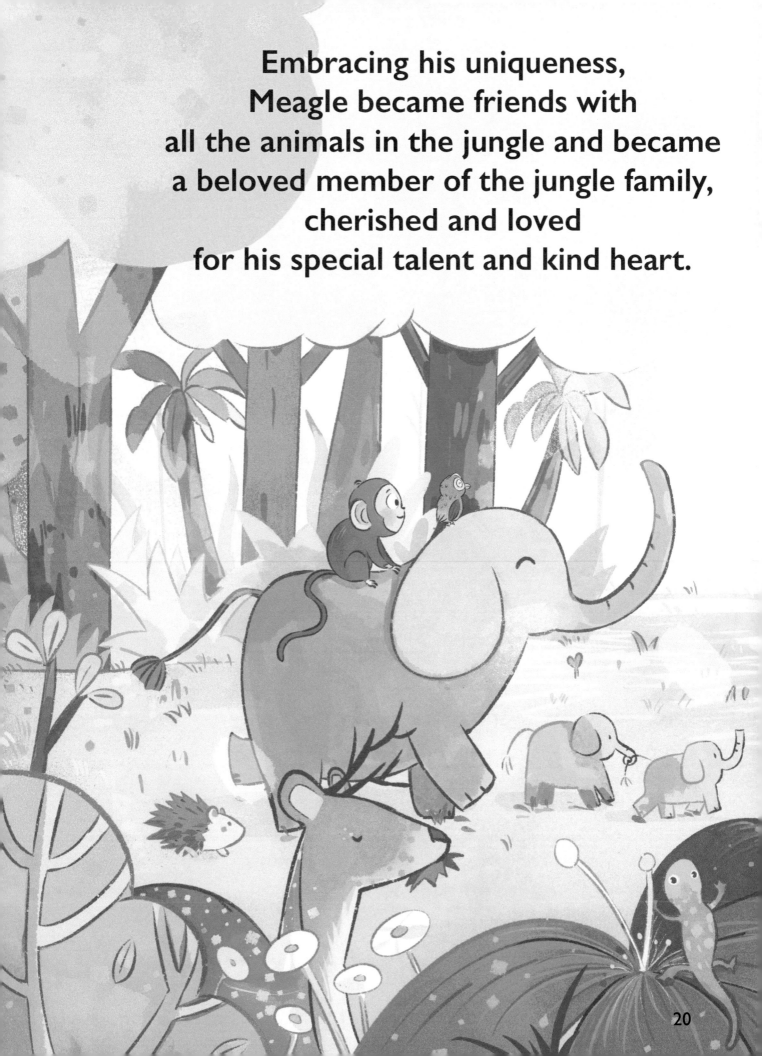

What makes Meagle different from the other monkeys?

1. He can fly.

2. He does not like fruits.

3. He is the same color as Piko

4. He is very sensitive to sounds.

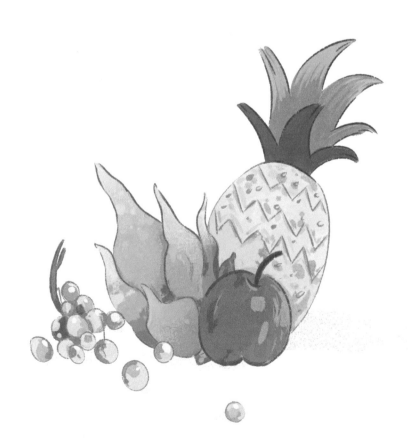

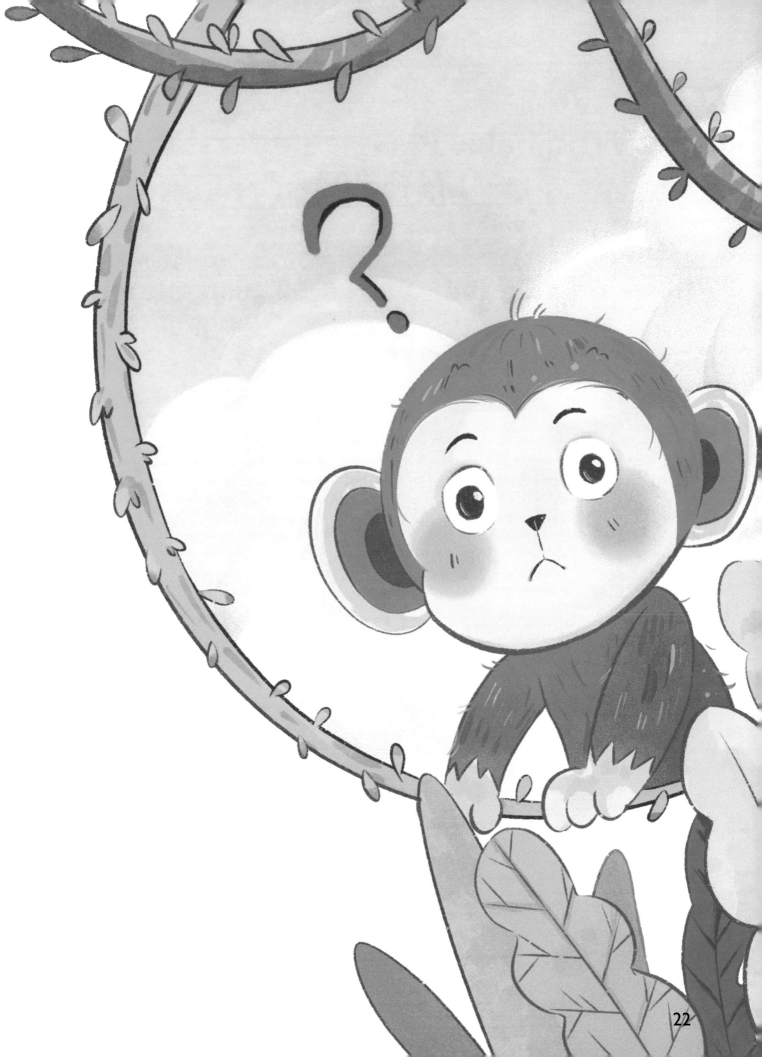

Who helps Meagle understand his feelings?

1. The fishes in the pond.

2. Piko, the wise owl.

3. A talking giraffe.

4. The roaring lion.

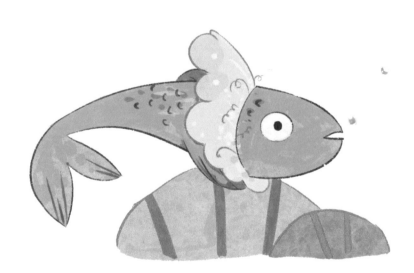

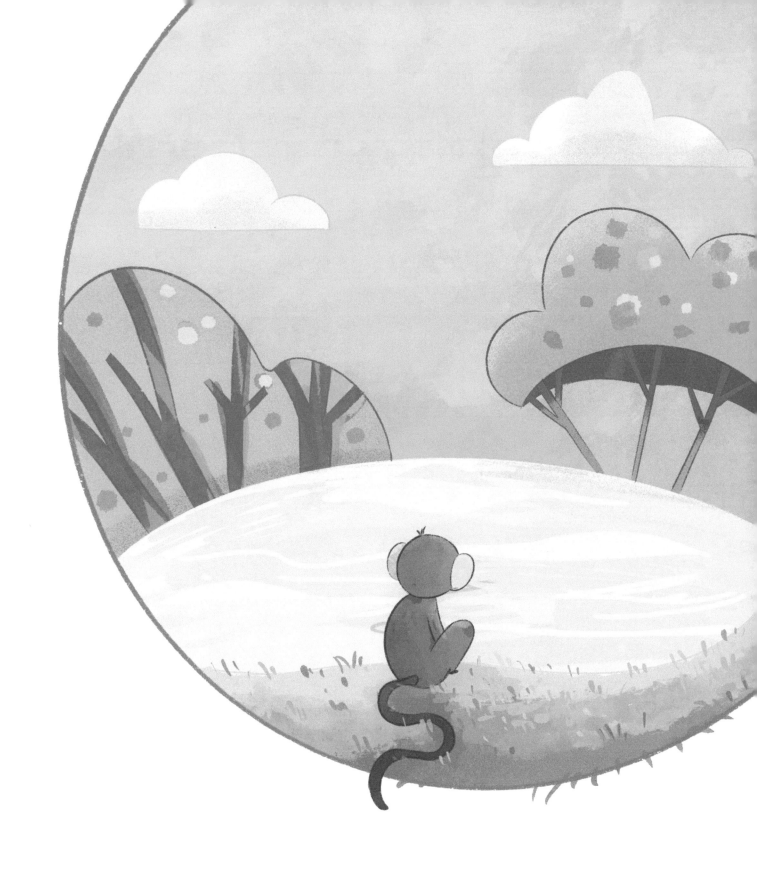

What does Meagle learn from Piko?

1. It is **OK** to be different.

2. Eat a lot of bananas.

3. Fly like Piko

4. To climb trees.

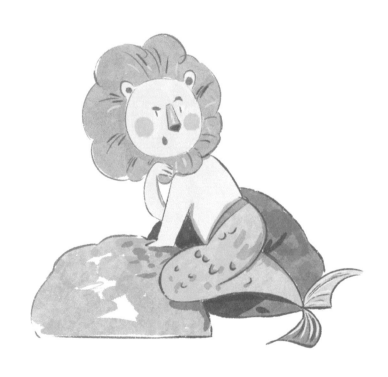

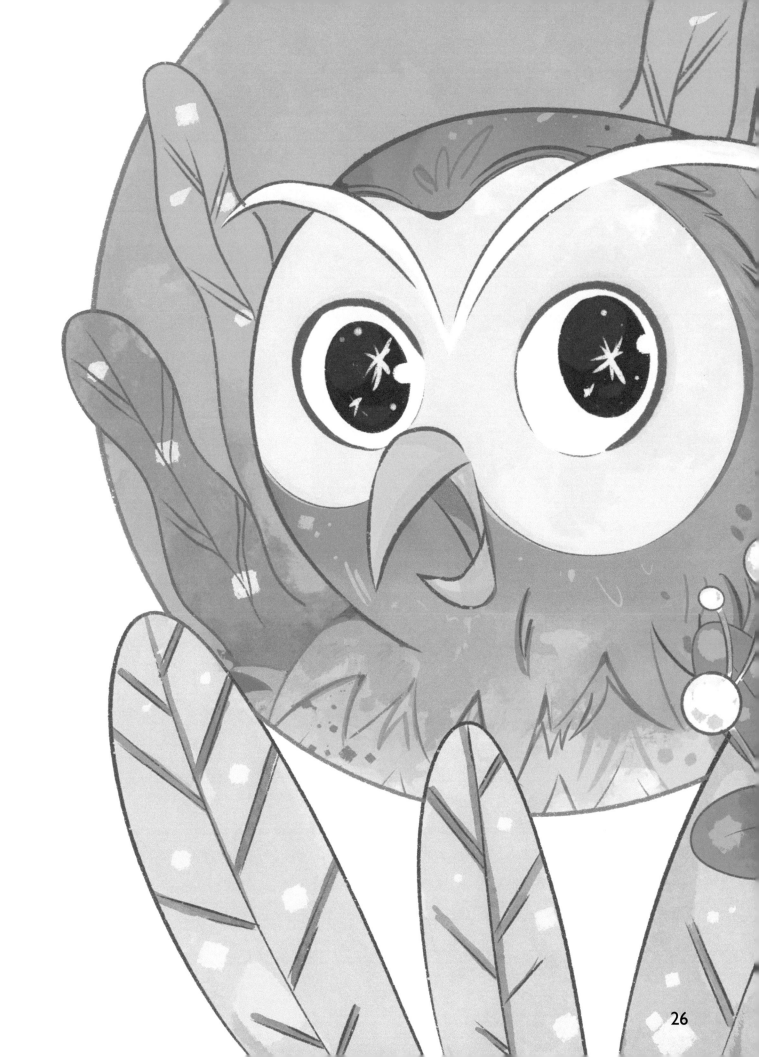